THE PERFECT MOBILE PHLEBOTOMY

& LAB PLAYBOOK

I0479287

BOSSLADI SANTRISE

THE PERFECT MOBILE PHLEBOTOMY & LAB PLAYBOOK

CHAPTER 1

From Concept to Reality

Hello and welcome. I'm excited to share with you my journey as a mobile phlebotomist and business owner. After working for over 10 years in the healthcare industry, I realized that there was a need for more convenient and personalized phlebotomy services. That's when I decided to start my own mobile phlebotomy business with value added services.

Through my experience, I've learned a lot about what it takes to build a successful business in this field, including the importance of having a strong brand, providing exceptional customer service, and staying up to date on the latest industry trends and technologies. Now, I'm passionate about sharing my knowledge and expertise with others who are interested in starting their own mobile phlebotomy businesses.

Whether you're a phlebotomist looking to break out on your own or an entrepreneur with *a passion for healthcare, my goal is to provide you with the tools and resources you need to succeed. So, let's get started and build a thriving mobile phlebotomy business together.*

There has never been a better time to get involved in the mobile phlebotomy industry. As the healthcare landscape continues to evolve, patients are increasingly seeking out more convenient and personalized care options. Mobile phlebotomy offers a unique solution to this demand, allowing patients to receive high-quality blood draw services in the comfort of their own homes or workplaces.

Jumping on the wave of mobile phlebotomy while it's still new offers a number of important advantages. For one, it allows you to establish yourself as an early player in a growing market, giving you a competitive edge over other providers. Additionally, by building a strong

brand and reputation early on, you can position yourself as a trusted leader in the industry, making it easier to attract new customers and build a loyal following.

Furthermore, the COVID-19 pandemic has highlighted the importance of mobile healthcare services, and many experts predict that this trend will continue well into the future.

By investing in mobile phlebotomy now, you can take advantage of this growing demand and build a thriving business that meets the evolving needs of patients and healthcare providers alike.

The mobile phlebotomy industry offers a wealth of opportunities for entrepreneurs and healthcare professionals alike. By jumping on the wave while it's still new, you can position yourself for long-term success and help shape the future of healthcare delivery.

Becoming an entrepreneur can have numerous benefits, including flexibility, control, financial potential, personal growth, and creating a footprint in the healthcare industry.

As an entrepreneur, you have the ability to set your own schedule and work on your own terms. This can provide greater work-life balance and allow you to pursue your passions and interests.

As a business owner, you have control over the direction of your company, including its products or services, marketing strategies, and overall vision. This can be empowering and rewarding, as you are able to see the results of your efforts.

While starting a business can be risky, it also has the potential to be highly profitable. As the owner, you can set your own pricing and determine your own income potential.

Building and running a business can provide opportunities for personal growth and development, such as building leadership skills, improving problem-solving abilities, and learning new things. As an entrepreneur, you have thepotential to make a positive impact on the world by providing a valuable product or service, creating jobs, and contributing to your community.

THE PERFECT MOBILE PHLEBOTOMY & LAB PLAYBOOK

CHAPTER 2
What Is A Mobile Phlebotomist?

A mobile phlebotomist is a healthcare professional who collects blood and other bodily fluids from patients at their homes, workplaces, or other locations outside of a traditional medical setting, such as a hospital or clinic.

Mobile phlebotomists are typically trained and certified in phlebotomy, which is the process of drawing blood for diagnostic or therapeutic purposes. They may also be trained to collect other types of samples, such as urine, saliva, or other bodily fluids, for laboratory testing.

The services provided by mobile phlebotomists can be particularly beneficial for patients who have difficulty traveling to a medical facility, such as those with mobility issues or busy schedules. Mobile phlebotomy services can also be convenient for patients who live in rural or remote areas, where access to healthcare services may be limited.

Quick replay, mobile phlebotomists play an

important role in ensuring that patients have access to necessary healthcare services, regardless of their location or mobility limitations.

CHAPTER 3

Why Should I Start A Mobile Phlebotomy & Lab Business?

A mobile phlebotomy business can be an excellent opportunity for those interested in healthcare, entrepreneurship, and flexibility. Starting a mobile phlebotomy business can be a viable and rewarding career option for several reasons.

Many people, especially those with mobility issues or busy schedules, find it difficult to visit a traditional laboratory for blood tests. Offering a mobile phlebotomy service brings the lab to them, making it more convenient for patients to receive necessary healthcare services.

As a mobile phlebotomist, you have the flexibility to choose your work hours and schedule appointments according to your availability. This allows you to balance your personal life and work commitments more easily.

A mobile phlebotomy business does not require a significant amount of capital investment. With a phlebotomy certification, you can start small and gradually build your business with minimal overhead costs.

Blood tests are an essential component of healthcare, and the demand for phlebotomy services is high. This means that there is always a steady stream of potential clients, especially in areas with a large aging population. As you build your reputation and client base, you can increase your fees, leading to a potentially lucrative income stream.

CHAPTER 4

Conduct Your Research

Conducting market research can help you to better understand your target audience, identify potential competitors, and develop effective marketing strategies for your mobile phlebotomy business. Here are some steps to conduct market research on mobile phlebotomy.

Start by defining the specific research objectives for your mobile phlebotomy business. This may include understanding the demographics and healthcare needs of your target audience, identifying potential competitors, and assessing demand for mobile phlebotomy services in your area.

Identify the specific demographic groups that are most likely to use your mobile phlebotomy services. This may include elderly patients, patients with mobility issues, and individuals with busy schedules.

Identify other mobile phlebotomy providers in your area and analyze their services, pricing, and marketing strategies. This can help you to identify areas of differentiation and competitive advantages for your business.

Collect data on your target audience and competition through a variety of sources, including surveys, online research, and focus groups. This can help you to better understand the needs and preferences of your target audience and develop effective marketing strategies.

Analyze the data you have collected to identify key insights and trends. Use this information to develop marketing strategies and business plans that are tailored to the needs of your target audience.

Quick replay, conducting market research can provide valuable insights into the needs and preferences of your target audience, the competitive landscape of the mobile phlebotomy industry, and potential marketing strategies for your business. It is important to use a variety of research methods and analyze the data carefully to develop effective marketing strategies and business plans.

CHAPTER 5

Income Potential

The income potential for becoming an independent mobile phlebotomist can vary depending on various factors such as geographic location, level of experience, demand for services, and the cost of living.

Independent mobile phlebotomists have the potential to earn a higher income than those working for an employer since they can set their own fees and have control over their workload. Independent mobile phlebotomists can also choose to specialize in serving particular niches, such as homebound patients or individuals requiring specialized tests, which can result in higher fees.

The income potential for independent mobile phlebotomists can also depend on the number of clients they serve and the frequency of their services. As the client base grows, and the number of services provided increases; the income potential may increase as well.

However, as an independent mobile phlebotomist, it is also important to consider the costs of running the business, such as purchasing equipment, marketing expenses, and transportation costs. These costs can affect the net income of the business.

Quick replay, the income potential for becoming an independent mobile phlebotomist can be influenced by various factors and can vary from one location to another. It is important to research the local market, set competitive pricing, and offer high-quality services to maximize income potential.

CHAPTER 6

Licenses And Certifications

The requirements for licenses or certifications to become an independent certified phlebotomist may vary depending on your location. In general, you may need to meet the following requirements.

Most states require that phlebotomists complete an accredited training program in phlebotomy. This may involve completing a certificate program, associate degree program, or other training program that includes both classroom instruction and hands-on training.

Many employers require phlebotomists to be certified by a recognized certification agency, such as the National Healthcare Association (NHA) or the American Society for Clinical Pathology (ASCP). To become certified, you may need to pass a certification exam and meet certain education and experience requirements.

Some states require phlebotomists to be licensed to practice. Licensure requirements may vary depending on your location, but may include passing an exam, meeting education and experience requirements, and paying a fee.

To maintain your certification or licensure, you may need to complete continuing education courses or meet other requirements to demonstrate ongoing competence in phlebotomy.

Quick replay, it is important to research the specific requirements in your location and consult with a professional organization or regulatory agency to ensure that you are meeting all of the necessary requirements to become an independent certified phlebotomist.

CHAPTER 7

Registered Or Certified Medical Assistant

Yes, you can be a certified or registered medical assistant and still own a mobile phlebotomy business. Being a certified medical assistant can provide you with the knowledge and skills necessary to perform phlebotomy, as well as other medical procedures. However, it is important to note that running a mobile phlebotomy business may require additional licenses or certifications, depending on your location.

Quick replay, it is important to research the specific requirements in your location and consult with a professional organization or regulatory agency to ensure that you are meeting all of the necessary requirements to operate your business legally and safely.

CHAPTER 8

Equipment, Supplies, & Resources

Using personal protective equipment (PPE) is important when operating a mobile phlebotomy business for several reasons.

Protection for yourself: PPE, such as gloves, masks, and face shields, can help protect you from exposure to bloodborne pathogens and other infectious diseases during the blood draw process.

Protection for your clients: Using PPE can help prevent the spread of infectious diseases from one client to another.

Compliance with regulations: OSHA and other regulatory agencies require healthcare professionals to use PPE when working with potentially infectious materials, including blood.

Using PPE can help demonstrate a commitment to providing safe and professional services to your clients.

As a mobile phlebotomist, you will need a variety of equipment and supplies to perform blood draws on your clients. Here is a list of some of the essential items:

Blood collection tubes: Blood collection tubes are used to collect and store blood samples. You will need a variety of different types of tubes depending on the tests that will be performed.

Needles and syringes: Needles and syringes are used to collect blood from your clients. It is important to have a range of sizes to accommodate different patients.

Alcohol swabs: Alcohol swabs are used to clean the skin before a blood draw to prevent infection.

Gloves: Gloves are essential for protecting both you and your clients during the blood draw process.

Bandages: Bandages are used to cover the puncture site after a blood draw to stop bleeding and prevent infection.

Tourniquet: A tourniquet is used to apply pressure to the arm to help locate a vein for the blood draw.

Blood pressure cuff: A blood pressure cuff is used to measure blood pressure, which can be important in certain cases.

Cooler with ice packs: A cooler with ice packs is essential for transporting collected blood samples to the laboratory for testing.

Mobile phlebotomy chair: A mobile phlebotomy chair can be helpful for providing a comfortable and safe space for your clients during the blood draw.

Mobile phlebotomy bag or case: A mobile phlebotomy bag or case is essential for *organizing and carrying all of your equipment and supplies during appointments.*

Medical waste disposal: You will need to properly dispose of medical waste, such as needles and other sharps, according to regulatory requirements.

Transportation: You will need reliable transportation to travel to different locations and provide mobile phlebotomy services.

It is important to regularly restock your supplies and keep them organized to ensure that you are prepared for each appointment. Additionally, it is important to comply with all relevant safety and sanitation guidelines to protect both you and your clients.

CHAPTER 9

Phomemo

Phomemo is a portable label printer that can be used to label blood samples in the mobile phlebotomy business.

Labels generated by Phomemo are clear and easy to read, which can help to improve accuracy and prevent errors when identifying blood samples. Using a label printer like Phomemo can help to give your mobile phlebotomy business a professional appearance, which can help to build trust with your clients.

Phomemo can help to save time by allowing you to quickly print labels on-site, rather than having to write them by hand or print them off-site. Phomemo is portable, which means you can easily bring it with you to different locations and use it on-site.

Phomemo allows for customization of labels, which means you can include specific *information such as the patient's name, date and time of collection, and any special instructions.*

Quick replay, using Phomemo to label blood samples can provide several benefits, including improved accuracy, a professional appearance, time savings, portability, and customization. It is important to ensure that you have the appropriate training and equipment to use Phomemo safely and effectively in your mobile phlebotomy business.

CHAPTER 10

Centrifuge Machine

Having a centrifuge machine is important for a mobile phlebotomy business. A centrifuge machine separates the different components of the blood, such as plasma, red blood cells, and platelets. This is important for certain tests that require specific components to be analyzed.

It helps to preserve the quality of the blood sample by preventing the blood from clotting and separating before it reaches the laboratory for testing. It can help to streamline the blood collection process and increase efficiency by allowing multiple samples to be processed at once. This machine helps to ensure the accuracy of test results by separating the blood components and providing a clear sample for testing. Having a centrifuge machine shows a level of professionalism and dedication to providing high-quality services to your clients.

CHAPTER 11

Additional Benefits of Using A Centrifuge Machine

Adding platelet-rich plasma (PRP), platelet-rich fibrin (PRf), and concentrated growth factors (CGf) to your mobile phlebotomy business can provide several benefits. Offering PRP, PRf, and CGf services can provide an additional revenue stream for your mobile phlebotomy business.

PRP, PRf, and CGf treatments have become increasingly popular in the healthcare industry due to their effectiveness in treating a variety of conditions, such as musculoskeletal injuries and hair loss. PRP, PRf, and CGf treatments are non-invasive and require minimal downtime, making them attractive to patients who are looking for less invasive treatments.

The cost of producing PRP, PRF, and CGF is relatively low, which can lead to higher profit margins compared to other healthcare services.

These treatments can help you to diversify your services and provide a more comprehensive range of treatments to your clients.

Quick replay, adding PRP, PRF, and CGF services to your mobile phlebotomy business can provide several benefits, including an additional revenue stream, increased demand, and the potential for higher profit margins. It is important to carefully evaluate the market demand and regulatory requirements before offering these treatments, and to ensure that you have the appropriate training and equipment to perform the treatments safely and effectively.

CHAPTER 12

Vein Finder- The Ultimate Goal Is 1 Stick

A vein finder is a handheld device that uses near-infrared light to detect veins under the skin. Here are some benefits of having a vein finder in your mobile phlebotomy business.

A vein finder can help to reduce the number of sticks required to locate a vein, which can improve patient comfort and reduce the risk of complications. Using a vein finder can help to locate veins quickly and accurately, which can increase the efficiency of phlebotomy procedures and reduce the time it takes to perform them. By reducing the number of sticks required to locate a vein, a vein finder can help to reduce the cost of supplies and equipment used in phlebotomy procedures.

It can help to improve the accuracy of venipuncture by locating veins that may be difficult to see or palpate. By improving patient comfort and reducing the risk of complications, a vein finder can help to enhance patient satisfaction and improve the overall patient experience.

Quick replay, having a vein finder in your mobile phlebotomy business can help to improve patient comfort, increase efficiency, reduce costs, improve accuracy, and enhance patient satisfaction. It is important to use the vein finder correctly and to receive proper training and certification before using it in your phlebotomy procedures.

CHAPTER 13

Resources For A Quick Refresher If You're New, Have Little Confidence Or Have Strayed Away From The Field

A Phlebotomy quick study guide and order of draw vertical badge card are two helpful tools for phlebotomists to improve their knowledge and accuracy during blood collection procedures. Both the guide and card are inexpensive and available for purchase on Amazon

The Phlebotomy quick study guide and order of draw vertical badge card provide a quick reference for phlebotomists to easily access important information such as order of draw, tube colors, and additives. By having a quick reference tool, phlebotomists can improve their accuracy and reduce the risk of errors during blood collection procedures. Using a quick study guide and order of draw badge can help phlebotomists work more efficiently by reducing the time it takes to look up information. These reference tools can help to boost phlebotomists' confidence and reduce anxiety during blood collection procedures. Using a quick study guide and order of draw badge demonstrates professionalism and a commitment to accuracy and safety during blood collection procedures. The Phlebotomy quick study guide and order of draw vertical badge card are small and portable, making it easy for phlebotomists to carry them around and have access to important information at all times.

Quick replay, purchasing a Phlebotomy quick study guide and order of draw vertical badge card can provide phlebotomists with a helpful and convenient tool to improve their knowledge and accuracy during blood collection procedures. It is important to use these tools in conjunction with proper training and certification to ensure the highest quality of care for patients.

CHAPTER 14

Establishing A Business Name, Mission And Vision Statement

Having a professional business name, mission statement, and vision statement is important for several reasons. It can help to establish a strong brand identity for your business, which can be important for attracting customers and building a loyal customer base. A clear mission statement and vision statement can help to communicate your business's purpose and values to potential customers, employees, and other stakeholders. Having a mission statement and vision statement can help to provide a sense of direction and purpose for your business, which can be helpful in guiding business decisions and setting goals.

These components can help to build trust with your customers by communicating your business's commitment to providing high-quality *services and upholding ethical standards. A clear mission and vision statement can help to motivate employees by providing a sense of purpose and direction for their work. A professional business name, mission statement, and vision statement can help to differentiate your business from competitors by communicating your unique strengths, values, and goals.*

Quick replay, having a professional business name, mission statement, and vision statement is important for establishing a strong brand identity, communicating your business's purpose and values, providing a sense of direction, building trust, motivating employees, and setting yourself apart from competitors. It is important to take the time to develop clear and concise statements that accurately reflect your business's goals and values.

CHAPTER 15

Business Registration

You will need to register your business and obtain any necessary licenses or permits, such as a state or local phlebotomy certification, to operate your mobile phlebotomy business legally. Creating a legal business typically involves several steps, which may vary depending on the type of business and the state or country where the business is being formed.

Choose a name that is unique, easy to remember, and not already in use by another business in your state. Check with your state's business registration office to make sure the name is available.

Choose a legal structure for your business, such as a sole proprietorship, partnership, limited liability company (LLC), or corporation. Each structure has its own legal and tax implications, so it's important to choose the one that best suits your business goals.

Register your business with your state's business registration office. This may involve filing articles of incorporation, articles of organization, or other legal documents, depending on the structure of your business.

Obtain any necessary permits and licenses for your business, such as a business license, zoning permit, or professional license.

Obtain a tax identification number (TIN) or employer identification number (EIN) from the Internal Revenue Service (IRS). This will be used for tax purposes, including paying taxes and hiring employees.

Open a separate bank account for your business to keep your personal finances separate from your business finances.

Obtain any necessary insurance for your business, such as liability insurance or workers' compensation insurance.

It is important to note that the process of creating a legal business can be complex, and it may be helpful to consult with a lawyer or accountant to ensure you are following all legal requirements and regulations.

CHAPTER 16

Obtain A Virtual Or Coworking Space Address

Using a virtual or coworking space address for home-based businesses can provide several benefits. Having a professional address, rather than a residential address, can help to create a more professional image for your business, which can be important for building trust with customers and clients. It helps to protect your privacy by keeping your home address confidential. This can be important for security reasons and to avoid unsolicited mail and visitors. A virtual or coworking space address can help to lend credibility to your business, especially if you are just starting out. It can show that you have a physical presence and a professional image, even if you are working from home. Many of these spaces offer additional services, such as mail forwarding, receptionist services, and meeting room rentals, which can be beneficial for home-based businesses that need access to these services but don't have the resources to provide them on their own.

Renting a virtual or coworking space address can be more cost-effective than renting a traditional office space, which can be important for small businesses with limited budgets. Using a virtual or coworking space address for a home-based business can provide several benefits, including a professional image, privacy, credibility, access to additional services, and cost savings.

You should consider obtaining professional and general liability insurance to protect your business from potential legal claims, such as malpractice or negligence.

You will need marketing materials, such as business cards, brochures, and a website, to promote your mobile phlebotomy services to potential clients.

You may need electronic health records (EHR) software to document patient information and ensure HIPAA compliance.

Operating a mobile phlebotomy business requires effective administrative resources to manage the day-to-day operations of your business. Here are some administration resources you will need as well.

You will need reliable scheduling software to manage your appointments and ensure that you can provide timely services to your clients.

You will need billing and payment software to generate invoices and process payments from your clients. This software can also help you to manage your finances and track revenue and expenses. You will need effective communication tools, such as email (HIPAA regulated), phone, fax or text messaging, to communicate with your clients and manage their needs.

You will need an inventory management system to track and manage your supplies and ensure that you have the necessary equipment *and*

supplies to perform your services.

CHAPTER 17
Business Management Software

HoneyBook is a business management software platform that offers a variety of tools and features to help small business owners manage their workflows, streamline their processes, and automate their business tasks.

HoneyBook offers a range of tools for managing client information, including contact information, contracts, invoices, and payments. This can help you to keep track of your clients and stay organized. HoneyBook automates your workflow, which can help to save time and increase efficiency. You can create templates for proposals, contracts, and other documents, and set up automated reminders for deadlines and follow-ups. HoneyBook provides tools for tracking your finances, including invoicing, payments, and expense tracking. This can help you to stay on top of your business finances and make informed decisions about your business. HoneyBook allows you to collaborate with clients and team members, which can help to streamline communication and increase productivity. You can share files, send messages, and assign tasks, all within the HoneyBook platform. This software offers a range of customization options, including branding and design, so you can personalize the platform to suit your business's needs and style.

Quick replay, HoneyBook can provide several benefits for small business owners, including client management, workflow automation, financial tracking, collaboration, and customization. It is important to evaluate your business's specific needs and goals before choosing a business management software platform like HoneyBook.

CHAPTER 18

Structuring Your Business

There are several ways to structure a business, each with its own advantages and disadvantages.

Sole proprietorship: A sole proprietorship is the simplest form of business structure, where an individual owns and operates the business on their own. The owner is personally liable for all debts and legal obligations of the business, but also has complete control over decision-making and business operations.

Partnership: A partnership is a business owned by two or more individuals who share the profits and losses of the business. Partnerships can be general, where all partners share equally in profits and losses, or limited, where one or more partners have limited liability.

Limited Liability Company (LLC): An LLC is a hybrid structure that combines the advantages of a partnership and a corporation. It offers personal liability protection for the owners, while still allowing them to maintain control over the business.

Corporation: A corporation is a legal entity that is separate from its owners, meaning that the owners are not personally liable for the debts and legal obligations of the business. Corporations can issue stocks, making it easier to raise capital and attract investors.

Cooperative: A cooperative is a business owned and controlled by its members, who share in the profits and decision-making. Cooperatives are often used in agriculture, retail, and other industries where a group of individuals have a common interest.

The choice of business structure will depend on factors such as the size of the business, the level of personal liability protection desired, and the tax implications of each structure. It is important to consult with a legal and financial professional when choosing the best structure for your business.

BOSSLADI SANTRISE

CHAPTER 19

Business Trust 101

Putting your business into a trust can provide several benefits, including:

Asset protection: Placing your business in a trust can help protect it from creditors or legal judgments, as the business assets are held separately from your personal assets.

Tax benefits: Depending on the type of trust, you may be able to take advantage of tax benefits such as reduced estate taxes or lower capital gains taxes.

Succession planning: Trusts can provide a way to plan for the transfer of ownership and management of the business after you pass away, ensuring that your business is passed on to the appropriate heirs or beneficiaries.

The process of putting your business into a trust will depend on the type of trust you choose and the specific requirements of your state.

Choose the type of trust: There are several types of trusts, including revocable and irrevocable trusts, A revocable trust, also known as a living trust, is a trust that can be changed or terminated by the trustor at any time during their lifetime. The trustor can transfer assets into the trust and name themselves as the trustee, giving them control over the assets during their lifetime. The trustor can also name one or more beneficiaries to receive the assets upon their death. The benefit of a revocable trust is that it allows the trustor to retain control over their assets during their lifetime, while also providing for the distribution of those assets after their death.

An irrevocable trust, on the other hand, is a trust that cannot be changed or terminated by the trustor once it has been created. Once assets are transferred into an irrevocable trust, they are no longer owned by the trustor and are instead owned by the trust. The trustor names a *trustee to manage the assets on behalf of one or more beneficiaries. The benefit of an irrevocable trust is that it can provide greater asset protection and estate tax benefits, as the assets are no longer considered part of the trustor's estate for tax purposes.*

The main difference between a revocable and irrevocable trust is the degree of control that the trustor retains over their assets. A revocable trust provides greater flexibility and control during the trustor's lifetime, while an irrevocable trust can provide greater asset protection and tax benefits.

Each has its own benefits and drawbacks. Consult with a legal professional to determine which type of trust is best for your business.

The trust agreement will outline the terms of the trust, including who will manage the trust, who the beneficiaries are, and how the trust assets will be distributed. Transfer ownership of your business to the trust, which may involve filing paperwork with your state and updating business registrations and licenses. Transfer business assets to the trust, which may include transferring ownership of real estate, equipment, and intellectual property.

Once the trust is established, it must be properly maintained, which may involve annual reporting requirements and other legal formalities. It is important to work with a legal and financial professional when setting up a trust for your business to ensure that it is done correctly and to maximize the benefits of the trust structure.

CHAPTER 20

Apply For EIN

An Employer Identification Number (EIN) is a unique nine-digit number assigned by the Internal Revenue Service (IRS) to businesses and other entities for tax identification purposes. You will need an EIN if you are starting a new business, hiring employees, operating as a partnership or corporation, or filing certain tax returns.

You can apply for an EIN online, by mail, fax, or telephone. The easiest and fastest way to apply is online through the IRS website. The EIN application will require you to provide information about your business, including your legal name, trade name, business address, type of business, number of employees, and other relevant information.

After filling out the application, submit it to the IRS. If applying online, you will receive your EIN immediately. If applying by mail, fax, or telephone, it may take several weeks to receive your EIN. Once you receive your EIN, use it to identify your business for tax purposes, such as on tax returns, employment tax forms, and other documents. It is important to note that there is no cost to apply for an EIN, and you only need one EIN per business entity.

CHAPTER 21

Services You Can Provide

As a mobile phlebotomist, you can offer a variety of services to your clients, including:

Blood draws for diagnostic tests: This is the primary service provided by mobile phlebotomists. You can collect blood samples from patients for laboratory tests to diagnose various conditions, such as diabetes, cholesterol levels, and infections.

Blood draws for therapeutic purposes: Some medical treatments require regular blood draws for therapeutic purposes, such as for chemotherapy, blood transfusions, or monitoring medication levels. Mobile phlebotomists can provide these services in the patient's home or other location.

Specimen collection: In addition to blood draws, mobile phlebotomists can collect other *types of specimens for laboratory testing, such as urine, saliva, or stool samples.*

Health screenings: Mobile phlebotomists can provide health screenings for conditions such as high blood pressure, cholesterol levels, and diabetes. These screenings can be useful for identifying potential health problems early on and developing treatment plans.

Vaccinations: Some mobile phlebotomists also offer vaccination services, such as flu shots or other immunizations.

As a mobile phlebotomist, you can provide a range of essential healthcare services that are convenient for patients who are unable to travel to a traditional medical setting.

CHAPTER 22

Locations You Can Serve

As a mobile phlebotomist, you can provide services in a variety of locations based on the needs of your clients.

Private homes: Many clients prefer the convenience of having blood draws done in the comfort of their own homes, especially if they have mobility issues or busy schedules.

Offices or workplaces: Business professionals may prefer to have blood draws done at their workplace to minimize time away from work.

Nursing homes or assisted living facilities: Elderly or disabled individuals may require blood draws but are unable to travel to a laboratory or medical facility, making mobile phlebotomy services a convenient option.

Hotels or resorts: Clients who are traveling may require blood draws for medical reasons, and mobile phlebotomy services can provide a convenient solution.

Doctor's offices or clinics: Mobile phlebotomists can provide services in a medical office or clinic setting, offering additional convenience for patients who are already receiving medical care.

Events or gatherings: Mobile phlebotomy services can also be offered at events, such as health fairs, wellness events, or community gatherings.

Mobile phlebotomists can service a variety of locations based on the needs of their clients, providing a convenient and efficient solution for blood draws and other specimen collections.

CHAPTER 23

Targeting Affluent Clientele & Areas

Targeting affluent clients and areas for your mobile phlebotomy services can help to increase your revenue and visibility in the industry.

Research the types of individuals or businesses that you want to target and network with other professionals in those industries. Attend events or join groups where these individuals or businesses are likely to be present and make connections.

Develop a marketing plan that targets the affluent clients and areas that you want to serve. Use social media, online directories, and other marketing channels to promote your services and highlight the benefits of using your mobile phlebotomy services.

Consider offering specialized services that are tailored to the needs of affluent clients. This may include offering expedited results, customized reports, or personalized service.

Partnering with other businesses in affluent areas can help to increase your visibility and reach. For example, you could partner with a concierge service or healthcare provider in a luxury hotel or resort to offer mobile phlebotomy services to their clients.

Word of mouth is a powerful marketing tool, especially in affluent circles. Providing exceptional service and going above and beyond to meet the needs of your clients can help to build a positive reputation and increase referrals.

Quick replay, targeting affluent clients and areas for your mobile phlebotomy services requires a strategic approach and a willingness to network and promote your services. By focusing on the needs of affluent clients and providing exceptional service, you can build a successful mobile phlebotomy business in these markets.

Targeting affluent clients and areas for your mobile phlebotomy services can have several benefits. Affluent clients may be willing to pay higher fees for the convenience and personalized service of mobile phlebotomy services, increasing your revenue potential.

Serving affluent clients and areas can increase your visibility and reputation in the industry, leading to more referrals and business opportunities. Targeting affluent clients and areas can provide access to a niche market that is underserved by traditional laboratory services, allowing you to differentiate yourself from competitors.

Affluent clients may require regular blood draws and specimen collections, providing opportunities for long-term relationships and recurring revenue.

Serving affluent clients and areas can provide networking opportunities with other professionals and businesses in related industries, leading to partnerships and collaborations.

Quick replay, targeting affluent clients and areas for your mobile phlebotomy services can lead to increased revenue, visibility, and reputation, as well as provide access to a niche market and networking opportunities. However, it is important to ensure that you are offering high-quality services and meeting the unique needs of affluent clients to maximize these benefits.

CHAPTER 24

Other Types of Patients

As a mobile phlebotomist, you can consider a wide range of individuals as potential patients for your business. Here are some examples of individuals who may benefit from mobile phlebotomy services.

Elderly or disabled individuals may have mobility issues or require specialized care, making it difficult for them to travel to a laboratory or medical facility. Mobile phlebotomy services can provide a convenient solution for collecting blood samples or other specimens in their homes or care facilities.

Business professionals may have busy schedules or limited availability, making it difficult for them to visit a laboratory or medical facility for blood tests. Mobile phlebotomy services can provide a convenient and time-saving option for collecting blood samples at their workplace or home.

Individuals with chronic illnesses, such as diabetes or kidney disease, may require regular blood tests or specimen collections to manage their condition.

Homebound individuals, such as those recovering from surgery or illness, may require blood tests or specimen collections but are unable to leave their homes. Mobile phlebotomy services can provide a safe and efficient option for collecting these samples in the comfort of their own homes.

Individuals in remote or rural areas may have limited access to healthcare facilities, making it difficult for them to receive blood tests or other medical services. Mobile phlebotomy services can provide a convenient and accessible option for collecting blood samples or other specimens in these areas.

Quick replay, there is a wide range of individuals who may benefit from mobile phlebotomy services, including those with *mobility*

issues, busy schedules, chronic illnesses, homebound individuals, and those in remote or rural areas. As a mobile phlebotomist, it is important to understand the needs of your potential patients and tailor your services to meet those needs.

CHAPTER 25

Generating Multiple Streams Of Income

There are several ways that a mobile phlebotomist can generate multiple streams of income.

Mobile phlebotomy services: The primary source of income for a mobile phlebotomist is offering phlebotomy services to clients. This can include but not limited to individuals, businesses, healthcare facilities, clinical study contracts, offering specialty kits, prp nano needling treatments, prenatal paternity testing, gender reveal testing as early 6 to 7 weeks of pregnancy, selling lab test and earning a commission, contracting with major sports teams, contracting with film studios, being a personal phlebotomist to celebrities and affiliate marketing. The possibilities are endless!

PRP, PRF, and CGF procedures: A mobile phlebotomist can offer additional services such as platelet-rich plasma (PRP), platelet-rich fibrin (PRF), and concentrated growth factors (CGF) procedures. These procedures involve using a patient's own blood to promote healing and can be used for cosmetic, orthopedic, and other medical purposes.

Consulting services: A mobile phlebotomist can offer consulting services to individuals or businesses looking to set up their own phlebotomy clinics. This can include advising on equipment and supplies, regulatory compliance, and best practices for patient care.

Education and training: A mobile phlebotomist can offer education and training services to individuals or groups interested in learning more about phlebotomy. This can include training for aspiring phlebotomists, continuing education for current phlebotomists, and workshops for healthcare professionals.

Product sales: A mobile phlebotomist can generate income by selling related products such *as phlebotomy supplies, medical equipment, or branded merchandise.*

CHAPTER 26

Therapeutic Phlebotomy

Therapeutic phlebotomy is a medical procedure that involves the removal of a specific amount of blood from a patient's body as a treatment for certain medical conditions. This is typically done using standard phlebotomy techniques, where a needle is inserted into a vein to collect blood.

Therapeutic phlebotomy is primarily used to treat medical conditions in which the body produces an excess of red blood cells, white blood cells, or iron. By removing a certain amount of blood, therapeutic phlebotomy can help reduce the levels of these substances in the body and alleviate symptoms associated with these conditions.

Some conditions that may benefit from therapeutic phlebotomy include:

Polycythemia vera: A condition in which the body produces too many red blood cells, which can lead to blood clots and other complications.

Hemochromatosis: A condition in which the body absorbs too much iron, leading to iron overload and potential organ damage.

Porphyria cutanea tarda: A rare condition that affects the skin and can cause blistering and sensitivity to sunlight.

Sickle cell disease: A genetic condition in which red blood cells are shaped abnormally and can cause pain, organ damage, and other complications.

Therapeutic phlebotomy is typically performed by a healthcare professional such as a phlebotomist, nurse, or physician. The procedure is generally safe, but it can cause side effects such as dizziness, fainting, or infection if not performed correctly.

CHAPTER 27

Professional Specimen Collector

The value proposition of becoming a certified drug and alcohol and DOT and Non-DOT professional specimen collector with your mobile phlebotomy business is that you can offer a comprehensive, highly specialized service to your clients. As a certified collector, you will be qualified to collect and handle urine samples for drug and alcohol testing for both DOT and non-DOT companies.

Having this certification can set your mobile phlebotomy business apart from competitors and demonstrate to potential clients that you have the necessary expertise to collect and handle specimens correctly. This can lead to more opportunities for business growth and potential revenue.

In addition to offering DOT and non-DOT specimen collection services, being a certified drug and alcohol collector can also provide additional revenue streams for your mobile phlebotomy business. Drug and alcohol testing is becoming increasingly important for many industries, and having a certified professional available to collect samples can make the process more efficient and streamlined for businesses.

Moreover, by providing both DOT and non-DOT drug and alcohol specimen collection services, your mobile phlebotomy business can offer a one-stop-shop solution for employers' drug and alcohol testing needs. This convenience can lead to more business opportunities and customer loyalty. Target Substance Abuse Professionals, Master Addiction Counselors, and Certified Associate Counselor-Alcohol and Alcohol (CAC-AD). Court orders for drug tests can include divorce, child custody cases, crime, and released on probation.

Quick replay, the value proposition of becoming a certified drug and alcohol DOT and non-DOT professional specimen collector with your mobile phlebotomy business is that you can offer a highly specialized, comprehensive service, *set yourself apart from competitors, expand your customer base, and potentially increase revenue and business growth opportunities.*

CHAPTER 28

Nano Needling

Nano needling with PRP centrifuging is a cosmetic procedure that combines the benefits of nano needling with the regenerative properties of platelet-rich plasma (PRP). The procedure involves drawing blood from the patient, spinning it in a centrifuge to separate the platelet-rich plasma, and then using a specialized device to perform the nano needling treatment with the PRP applied topically. Some of the common uses of nano needling with PRP centrifuging include:

Anti-aging: Nano needling with PRP can help improve the appearance of fine lines, wrinkles, and other signs of aging by stimulating collagen production and skin regeneration.

Acne scars: The treatment can help reduce the appearance of acne scars by promoting collagen production and encouraging the growth of new, healthy skin cells.

73

Hyperpigmentation: Nano needling with PRP can also help reduce hyperpigmentation, such as age spots and sunspots, by encouraging the skin to produce new cells.

Hair loss: The procedure can also be used to promote hair growth and improve the appearance of thinning hair.

The effectiveness of nano needling with PRP can vary depending on individual factors, such as age, skin type, and the severity of the skin condition being treated. Generally, patients can expect to see results within 2-3 weeks of the treatment, with continued improvement over several months. Recovery time can vary depending on the individual, but most patients can return to their normal activities immediately after the procedure with only minor redness and swelling.

Adding nano needling with PRP centrifuging to your business can help you offer a wider range of services to your clients, which can help attract new customers and increase revenue. The combination of nano needling with

PRP can provide more dramatic and longer-lasting results than either procedure alone.

As a more advanced and specialized procedure, nano needling with PRP centrifuging can command higher prices than standard nano needling. By offering a range of services, you can increase your client satisfaction and build long-term relationships with your clients.

Quick replay, nano needling with PRP centrifuging is a safe and effective procedure that can help improve a variety of skin and hair conditions. As with any cosmetic procedure, it's important to ensure that you have the necessary training and expertise before offering this service to your clients.

CHAPTER 29

Affiliate Marketing

Affiliate marketing can be a great way to generate additional income for your mobile phlebotomy business. Look for affiliate programs that are relevant to your business, such as medical supply companies or health and wellness products. Research their commission rates, payment methods, and any other requirements for joining.

Select products that are relevant to your audience and that you believe in. You can promote these products on your website, social media platforms, or through email marketing. Develop content that promotes the affiliate products and provides value to your audience. This can include product reviews, tutorials, and guides.

Use various marketing channels to promote the affiliate products, such as social media, email marketing, and paid advertising.

Be transparent about your affiliate relationships. Use tracking tools to monitor your affiliate sales and optimize your campaigns based on performance. Continually test and refine your strategies to improve your results.

Affiliate marketing can be a lucrative and scalable way to generate additional income for your mobile phlebotomy business. As with any business strategy, it's important to do your research and ensure that you are promoting products that align with your values and are relevant to your audience.

Quick replay, a mobile phlebotomist can generate multiple streams of income by offering a range of services and products related to phlebotomy, consulting, education, and product sales. It is important to ensure that any additional services or products offered are in compliance with relevant regulations and guidelines.

CHAPTER 30

Maximize Your Business

Providing excellent customer service can help you to build a loyal customer base and generate positive word-of-mouth referrals. This can be especially important in the healthcare industry, where patients may be anxious or uncomfortable.

Consider expanding your services to include additional healthcare services, such as wellness screenings or flu shots. This can help you to provide more comprehensive care for your clients and increase your revenue.

Build partnerships with other healthcare providers, such as doctors, clinics, and laboratories, to expand your network and provide additional services to your clients.

Develop a strong online presence through websites and social media channels, such as

Facebook and Instagram. This can help you to reach a wider audience and promote your services. Use technology to streamline your business operations, such as scheduling and billing software. This can help you to save time and improve efficiency.

Focus on marketing your business through targeted advertising, search engine optimization (SEO), and content marketing. This can help you to attract new clients and build your brand. Stay up to date with industry trends and best practices, such as changes to healthcare regulations and advancements in medical technology. This can help you to stay competitive and provide the best possible care for your clients. By implementing these tips, you can maximize your business as a mobile phlebotomist and achieve your business goals.

CHAPTER 31

Online Visibility

Listing your business on Google and optimizing your website for search engines can help to increase your visibility online. This can make it easier for potential clients to find your business and learn more about your services. A well-designed and optimized website can improve the credibility of your mobile phlebotomy business. This can help to build trust with potential clients and increase the likelihood of them choosing your services over competitors.

By optimizing your website for search engines, you can improve your ranking on search engine results pages (SERPs) and potentially outrank competitors. This can give you a competitive advantage in the market and increase the likelihood of attracting new clients. SEO optimization can help you to target specific keywords and phrases related to your mobile phlebotomy business. This can help you to attract potential clients who are specifically searching for the services you offer. Listing your business on Google and optimizing your website for search engines can be a cost-effective way to market your mobile phlebotomy business. Compared to traditional marketing methods, such as print ads or billboards, SEO optimization can provide a higher return on investment.

Quick replay, listing your business on Google and optimizing your website for search engines can provide several benefits for your mobile phlebotomy business, including increased visibility, improved credibility, a competitive advantage, better targeting, and cost-effective marketing. By investing in these strategies, you can improve the online presence of your business and attract new clients to grow your business.

CHAPTER 32

The Process Of Listing Your Business On Google

Adding your business to Google can help improve your online presence and make it easier for potential customers to find you. Here are the steps to add your business on Google:

Go to the Google My Business website: https://www.google.com/business/ and sign in with your Google account. If you don't have a Google account, you'll need to create one.

Enter your business name, address, phone number, and website URL. You will also need to choose a category that best describes your business. Google will ask you to verify your business by mail, phone, or email. The verification process can take up to two weeks.

Once your business is verified, you can optimize your listing by adding photos, business hours, and other details about your business.

You can also respond to customer reviews and monitor your online reputation. Once you have optimized your listing, click the "Publish" button to make your listing live on Google.

It is important to keep your business information up to date on Google and monitor your listing for accuracy and customer feedback. Regularly updating your listing can help improve your online visibility and attract more customers to your business.

CHAPTER 33

Different Marketing Channels

Marketing your mobile phlebotomy lab with value-added services through various channels, including social media, blogging, business listings, pay per click (PPC) ads, and industry associations.

By utilizing multiple marketing channels, you can increase brand awareness and reach a wider audience, potentially generating more leads and increasing sales. Each marketing channel offers unique targeting options that allow you to reach specific demographics or interests. For example, social media advertising can target users based on their interests, while PPC ads can target specific keywords or search terms. Creating blog content and business listings can improve your website's search engine rankings, making it more visible to potential customers who are searching for your services.

Many digital marketing channels, such as social media and blogging, can be cost-effective, allowing you to reach a large audience without breaking the bank.

By highlighting your value-added services, such as mobile phlebotomy, you can differentiate your business from competitors and provide a unique selling point that can attract new customers. Joining industry associations can provide networking opportunities, access to industry-specific resources, and potential referrals from other members.

Quick replay, utilizing multiple marketing channels to promote your mobile phlebotomy lab with value-added services can help increase brand awareness, generate leads, and differentiate your business from competitors, ultimately leading to increased revenue and business growth.

CHAPTER 34

Becoming HIPAA & OSHA Certified

HIPAA (Health Insurance Portability and Accountability Act) is a federal law that regulates the use and disclosure of personal health information (PHI). As a mobile phlebotomist, you will have access to PHI when collecting blood samples and performing other specimen collections. Therefore, it is important to be HIPAA certified to ensure that you are protecting patient privacy and complying with the law.

Here are some reasons why you need to be HIPAA certified with your mobile phlebotomy business.

HIPAA is a federal law that applies to all healthcare providers, including mobile phlebotomists. Failure to comply with HIPAA regulations can result in severe penalties and fines. HIPAA regulations require that patient *privacy is protected, including the use and disclosure of PHI. As a mobile phlebotomist, you will have access to PHI and must take steps to ensure that it is not disclosed improperly. HIPAA compliance can help to build trust with clients by demonstrating that you take their privacy seriously and are committed to protecting their personal health information. HIPAA compliance can help to prevent data breaches and minimize the risk of PHI being accessed by unauthorized individuals. HIPAA compliance is an industry standard for all healthcare providers, including mobile phlebotomists. Being HIPAA certified can help you to meet these standards and demonstrate your professionalism and commitment to the highest ethical standards.*

Quick replay, being HIPAA certified with your mobile phlebotomy business is essential to protect patient privacy, comply with legal requirements, build trust with clients, prevent data breaches, and meet industry standards.

As a mobile phlebotomist, you are required to comply with OSHA (Occupational Safety and Health Administration) standards to ensure a safe work environment. While OSHA certification is not mandatory for phlebotomists, it is highly recommended and may be required by some employers. OSHA provides training and certification programs for various industries, including healthcare, that cover topics such as bloodborne pathogens, personal protective equipment (PPE), and hazard communication.

You will likely be working in a variety of settings, including private homes and businesses, which may have unique safety hazards that you need to be aware of. By obtaining OSHA certification, you will gain knowledge and skills in identifying and minimizing workplace hazards, handling hazardous materials, and using PPE to protect yourself and your clients.

Additionally, OSHA compliance can help you establish credibility with potential clients and demonstrate a commitment to safety and quality of care. OSHA certification can also be beneficial if you plan to work with healthcare facilities or other employers who require it as a condition of employment.

Quick replay, while OSHA certification is not required to work as a mobile phlebotomist, it can be highly beneficial in ensuring a safe work environment and demonstrating a commitment to safety and quality of care.

CHAPTER 35

Am I Required To Have A Medical Director?

The requirement for a medical director for a mobile phlebotomy business may vary depending on the state in which you operate. However, it is common for mobile phlebotomy businesses to have a medical director to oversee clinical practices and ensure compliance with regulatory requirements.

In some states, it may be a requirement to have a medical director for your mobile phlebotomy business. For example, in California, mobile phlebotomy businesses are required to have a licensed physician or nurse practitioner as a medical director. Other states may require that the medical director is a licensed physician or a licensed healthcare provider with specific training in phlebotomy.

Even if it is not a legal requirement in your state, having a medical director can provide many benefits for your mobile phlebotomy business. A medical director can provide oversight of clinical practices, ensure compliance with regulatory requirements, provide guidance on medical protocols, and advise on quality control measures. A medical director can also serve as a liaison between your business and other healthcare providers, helping to build relationships and referrals.

Quick replay, while the requirement for a medical director for a mobile phlebotomy business may vary by state, having a medical director can provide many benefits for your business, including improved clinical oversight and compliance with regulatory requirements. It is recommended to consult with your state's regulatory agencies and seek legal advice to determine the specific requirements for your mobile phlebotomy business.

CHAPTER 36
CLIA Waiver & NPI

In the United States, a mobile phlebotomy business may need a National Provider Identifier (NPI) number and/or a Clinical Laboratory Improvement Amendments (CLIA) waiver, depending on the services offered.

An NPI number is a unique identifier assigned to healthcare providers by the Centers for Medicare and Medicaid Services (CMS). If your mobile phlebotomy business is providing services that are reimbursable by Medicare, Medicaid, or private insurance, you may need an NPI number. The NPI number is used to identify healthcare providers in electronic transactions and on claim forms.

A CLIA waiver is a certificate that allows a laboratory to perform simple tests, known as waived tests, without meeting all of the requirements of the Clinical Laboratory Improvement Amendments (CLIA) regulations. If *your mobile phlebotomy business is performing waived tests, such as fingerstick blood glucose testing, rapid influenza tests, blood glucose monitors, strep A tests, Hemoglobin A1c tests, urine dipstick tests, fecal occult blood tests, and so many more, you may need a CLIA waiver.*

It is important to note that the requirements for NPI numbers and CLIA waivers may vary by state and by the services offered. It is recommended that you consult with your state's health department and/or the CMS to determine whether an NPI number and/or CLIA waiver is required for your mobile phlebotomy business.

CHAPTER 37
CMS & EDI Registration

The Electronic Data Interchange (EDI) is a system used by the Centers for Medicare & Medicaid Services (CMS) to process claims and payments electronically. The Provider Enrollment, Chain, and Ownership System (PECOS) is an online system used to enroll healthcare providers and suppliers in the Medicare program.

If you have not already done so, you will need to enroll in the Medicare program. This can be done through the PECOS system.

You will need to obtain a National Provider Identifier (NPI) number, which is a unique identifier assigned to healthcare providers by CMS. You can obtain an NPI number through the National Plan and Provider Enumeration System (NPPES).

You will need to enroll in EDI to process claims and payments electronically. You can do this through the CMS Enterprise Portal.

A clearinghouse is a third-party entity that helps to process electronic claims and payments. You will need to choose a clearinghouse and sign up for their services. Once you are set up with EDI and a clearinghouse, you will need to test your system to ensure that it is working properly.

It is important to note that the process of getting set up to take payments from CMS can be complex and time-consuming. You may want to consider working with a healthcare consultant or billing service to help guide you through the process.

CHAPTER 38

Contracting With Private Insurance Companies

To contract with private insurance companies for reimbursement as a mobile phlebotomy business, you will need to follow these steps.

Many private insurance companies require healthcare providers to be licensed and certified in their respective states. Make sure that you have all of the necessary licensure and certification to provide phlebotomy services in your state.

You will need to obtain a National Provider Identifier (NPI) number, which is a unique identifier assigned to healthcare providers by the Centers for Medicare and Medicaid Services (CMS). You can obtain an NPI number through the National

Plan and Provider Enumeration System (NPPES).

Private insurance companies often require healthcare providers to carry malpractice insurance. Make sure that you have the appropriate level of malpractice insurance for your mobile phlebotomy business.

Research private insurance companies in your area to determine which ones are the best fit for your mobile phlebotomy business. Contact them to find out their specific requirements for contracting with healthcare providers.

Once you have identified insurance companies that you want to contract with, submit a provider application to each of them. The application will require you to provide information about your business, including your NPI number, malpractice insurance, and other relevant information.

After your provider application is accepted, you will need to negotiate rates with *the insurance company. Make sure that you understand the reimbursement rates for the services that you provide and negotiate rates that are fair and reasonable.*

Quick replay, contracting with private insurance companies for reimbursement as a mobile phlebotomy business can be a complex process. It is important to do your research, understand the requirements of the insurance companies, and negotiate fair and reasonable rates. You may want to consider working with a healthcare consultant or billing service to help guide you through the process.

CHAPTER 39

Business Banking & Separate Operating Accounts

Why is it important to have an income account, expense or operating account, payroll account, and tax or saving account for my business at the same bank?

Income account- Having a separate income account can make it easier to track your business's revenue and monitor your financial performance. You'll use this account for cash and credit card deposits. You'll also need these account statements for any loans or credit applications. This account should never be negative.

Expense or Operating Account- This account will have a check card and business checks to pay for your business operating expenses. Money will be transferred from the income account into your expenses or operating account. A separate expense or operating account can make it easier to generate financial reports and share them with stakeholders, such as investors or lenders. Also, this account can provide legal protection by separating your business's expenses from your personal finances. This can help to protect your personal assets in case of legal disputes or bankruptcy.

Payroll- Having a separate payroll account for your business can provide several benefits. Having a separate payroll account can make it easier to manage your payroll and ensure that your employees are paid accurately and on time. This can help to avoid errors and reduce the risk of legal or financial issues. Having a separate payroll account can make it easier to keep accurate records of your payroll expenses and track employee compensation. This can help you to comply with legal and regulatory requirements and simplify tax filing. Having a separate payroll account can make it easier to manage your cash flow and ensure that you have enough funds to cover payroll expenses. This can help to avoid cash flow challenges and ensure that your business remains financially stable. A separate payroll account can help you to comply with legal and regulatory requirements related to payroll, such as tax withholding and reporting. This can help to avoid legal or financial penalties and ensure that you are operating your business in a compliant manner. A separate payroll account can provide increased security for your business and your employees. This is because you can monitor your payroll expenses and quickly detect any fraudulent activity or errors.

Taxes or Savings Account-Having a separate savings account for your business can provide several benefits, including:

Emergency fund- A business savings account can serve as an emergency fund that you can tap into in case of unexpected expenses or cash flow challenges. Having a savings account can help to ensure that your business is prepared for unexpected events and can weather financial challenges. A business savings account can be used to save for future business opportunities or investments. For example, you may want to save for a new piece of equipment, expand your business, or invest in marketing. Having a savings account can help you to achieve these goals and grow your business. A business savings account can be used to set aside funds for tax payments or other financial obligations. This can help you to plan for these expenses and avoid cash flow challenges. Business savings accounts often offer higher interest rates than traditional savings accounts. This can help your business to earn more money from its savings and improve overall financial performance. A separate savings account can make it easier to manage your business finances and keep track of your savings. This can help you to make informed decisions about your business and improve financial management.

Having multiple accounts for your business at the same bank can provide several benefits as well. Having all of your business accounts at the same bank can make it easier to manage your finances and avoid the need to transfer funds between multiple banks. This can save time and reduce the risk of errors or delays. Separate accounts for income, expenses, payroll, and taxes can make it easier to manage your cash flow and ensure that you have enough funds to cover expenses and taxes. This can help to avoid cash flow challenges and ensure that your business remains financially stable. Having separate accounts for income, expenses, payroll, and taxes can make it easier to track and report on your business finances. This can help you to understand your financial performance and make informed decisions about your business. It's easier to set aside funds for taxes and ensure that you are complying with tax regulations. This can help to simplify the tax filing process and avoid penalties or legal issues. Business accounts at the same bank can provide increased security and reduce the risk of fraud or identity theft. This is because you can monitor all of your accounts in one place and quickly detect any suspicious activity.

Quick replay, having multiple accounts for your business at the same bank can provide many benefits, including convenience, improved cash flow management, improved financial reporting, simplified tax filing, and increased security. It is important to consult with a *financial advisor or accountant to determine the best approach for managing your business finances and ensure that you are complying with all legal and regulatory requirements.*

Having separate accounts for your business can make it easier to budget for business expenses and revenue. This can help you to manage cash flow effectively and avoid financial challenges. It helps to improve the professionalism of your business. This can help to build trust with clients and stakeholders and improve the reputation of your business.

Quick replay, having separate accounts for your business can provide many benefits, including legal protection, tax compliance, improved financial management, better budgeting, and improved professionalism. It is important to consult with a financial advisor or accountant to determine the best approach for managing your business finances and ensure that you are complying with all legal and regulatory requirements.

CHAPTER 40

Creating A Business Plan

A business plan can help you to define your business goals and strategies and identify the steps you need to take to achieve them. This can help to ensure that you are on the right track and making progress towards your desired outcomes.

If you plan to seek financing or investment for your business, a business plan can be an essential tool for demonstrating the potential of your business and your ability to achieve your goals. A well-written business plan can help to attract investors or lenders and secure the funding you need to start or grow your business. A business plan can help you to identify potential challenges that may arise as you start or grow your business. This can help you to prepare for these challenges and develop strategies for overcoming them. It can serve as a roadmap for your business, outlining the steps you need to take to achieve your goals and track your progress. This can help you to stay focused and motivated as you work towards building a successful business.

It can help you to make informed decisions about your business, by providing you with a clear understanding of your goals, strategies, and financial projections. This can help you to prioritize your actions and allocate resources effectively.

Quick replay, having a business plan for your mobile phlebotomy business can provide many benefits, including clarifying your goals and strategies, attracting investors or lenders, identifying potential challenges, providing a roadmap for success, and improving your decision-making. It is important to consult with a business advisor or mentor to develop a comprehensive business plan that addresses all aspects of your business and sets you up for success.

CHAPTER 41

Adjusting Your Mindset

Shifting from an employee mindset to a business owner and employer mindset can be challenging, but it is an essential step in building a successful business. As a business owner and employer, you are responsible for making decisions that impact the success of your business and the well-being of your employees. Embrace this new role and take ownership of your business. Develop a clear vision for your business and create a strategy to achieve your goals. This may involve setting short-term and long-term goals, identifying target markets, and creating a plan for marketing and sales.

Starting and running a business can be challenging, so seek advice and support from mentors, advisors, or other business owners who have experience in your industry. As an employer, you are responsible for hiring and managing employees. Build a strong team by hiring people who share your values and work ethic and provide them with the training and support they need to succeed. As a business owner, you are responsible for managing your finances and ensuring that your business remains profitable. Develop a budget, track your expenses and revenue, and seek advice from financial professionals if necessary.

Effective communication is essential in any business, so prioritize communication with your employees, customers, and other stakeholders. Listen to feedback and make adjustments as necessary to improve your business.

Quick replay, shifting from an employee mindset to a business owner and employer mindset requires a shift in mindset and approach. Embrace your new role, develop a clear vision and strategy, seek advice and support, build a strong team, manage your finances, and prioritize communication to set yourself up for success as a business owner and employer.

CHAPTER 42

Hiring Employees

Determine what positions you need to fill and what skills and qualifications you are looking for in candidates. Create a job description that outlines the responsibilities and qualifications for the position, as well as any necessary certifications or licenses.

Advertise the position through job postings, networking, and referrals. Consider posting on job boards or working with a staffing agency to find qualified candidates. Review resumes and conduct initial phone screenings to assess candidates' qualifications and interest in the position. Conduct in-person or virtual interviews with qualified candidates to assess their skills, experience, and fit for the position.

Conduct background checks and verify references to ensure candidates have the necessary qualifications and a history of good work performance. Once you have identified a qualified candidate, make a job offer that includes details about the position, salary, and benefits.

Provide comprehensive training and onboarding to ensure that the new employee is prepared to work effectively and safely. Ensure that you are complying with all legal requirements related to employment, including wage and hour laws, taxes, and workers' compensation insurance.

Remember that hiring employees can be a complex process, and it may be beneficial to work with an HR consultant or employment attorney to ensure that you are complying with all legal requirements and best practices.

CHAPTER 43

Hiring Independing Contractors

When hiring independent contractors for your mobile phlebotomy business, be clear about what you expect from the contractor, including the services they will provide, the hours they will work, and any other requirements or expectations.

Clearly communicate your expectations regarding professionalism, communication, and other important aspects of the job. Make sure the contractor understands their responsibilities and what is expected of them. Before hiring a contractor, conduct a background check and verify their credentials, including their phlebotomy certification and any necessary licenses or permits.

Provide proper training and support to ensure the contractor is equipped to provide high-quality services and adhere to your company's policies and procedures. Establish a contract that outlines the terms of the engagement, including the scope of work, compensation, and any other relevant details. Maintain open and regular communication with the contractor to ensure any issues or concerns are addressed promptly. Regularly evaluate the contractor's performance to ensure they are meeting expectations and providing high-quality services.

By following these best practices, you can build a successful working relationship with your independent contractor and ensure the continued success of your mobile phlebotomy business.

CHAPTER 44

Business Franchise

Creating a franchise for your mobile phlebotomy business can be a complex and time-consuming process. Before creating a franchise, you need to develop a strong brand identity that includes a clear mission, values, and business model. This will help you attract potential franchisees and ensure consistency across all locations.

Develop a business model that is scalable and can be easily replicated across multiple locations. This may include developing systems for training, support, and operations. Develop a franchise agreement that outlines the terms and conditions of the franchise relationship, including fees, royalties, and support services.

You will need to register your franchise with the Federal Trade Commission (FTC) and follow their guidelines for disclosure and *advertising. Once your franchise model is established, you can begin recruiting franchisees who share your vision and are willing to invest in your business. Provide comprehensive training and ongoing support to ensure that franchisees are successful and represent your brand well.*

Remember that creating a franchise is a complex and regulated process, and it may be beneficial to work with a franchise consultant or attorney who can guide you through the process and ensure that you are complying with all legal requirements.

CHAPTER 45

Interview Questions

When hiring mobile phlebotomists, here are some interview questions you may consider asking:

What is your phlebotomy experience?

What is your certification and what was involved in the training?

Have you worked with any specific populations or age groups?

Do you have experience working as a mobile phlebotomist?

Can you describe your process for preparing and transporting equipment and supplies to different locations?

How do you ensure patient confidentiality and compliance with HIPAA regulations while working in patients' homes or workplaces?

Can you describe a time when you had to manage a difficult patient? How did you handle the situation?

How do you stay up to date on industry best practices and new technologies?

What is your availability to work on a flexible schedule?

How would you ensure high-quality customer service and patient satisfaction?

Remember to tailor your questions to your specific business needs and to ask follow-up questions as necessary to ensure you are getting a clear understanding of the candidate's skills and experience.

CHAPTER 46

Establishing Business Credit

Building business credit can be an important step in establishing and growing your business. Before you can start building business credit, you need to establish your business as a separate entity from your personal finances. This may involve incorporating your business or obtaining a business license.

Opening a separate bank account for your business can help you to track your finances and build a credit history. Applying for a business credit card can help you to build credit by making regular payments on your account. Working with suppliers who report to credit bureaus can help to build your credit history by demonstrating that you are a responsible borrower.

Paying your bills on time is an important factor in building credit. Late payments can *negatively impact your credit score and make it more difficult to obtain credit in the future. Regularly monitoring your credit score can help you to identify areas where you need to improve and track your progress over time. As your business credit history improves, you may be able to apply for loans or lines of credit to help you grow your business.*

It is important to note that building business credit takes time and effort. It may take several years to establish a strong credit history, so it is important to be patient and persistent in your efforts to build credit. Additionally, it is important to maintain good financial practices, such as paying bills on time and keeping debt levels low, in order to maintain and improve your credit score.

Shorten those years by using this link for step-by-step details to build your business credit <u>How To Build Your Business Credit Fast | Nav</u> *or the website* https://www.nav.com/resource/how-to-establish-business-credit/

CHAPTER 47

Resources To Find Specialty Labs

ThomasNet is an online platform that connects buyers and suppliers in a wide range of industries, including healthcare. ThomasNet can help you to reach a large network of potential clients in the healthcare industry, including hospitals, clinics, and laboratories. Listing your mobile phlebotomy business on ThomasNet can increase your visibility and help you to stand out from competitors in your area.

ThomasNet allows you to target your marketing efforts to specific industries, regions, or types of businesses, which can help you to connect with potential clients who are most likely to be interested in your services. Being listed on ThomasNet can help to establish your business as a credible and trustworthy provider of mobile phlebotomy services. Many companies and organizations are seeking to diversify their supplier base, and listing your business on

ThomasNet can help you to connect with clients who are looking for diverse suppliers.

In the search bar enter medical testing laboratories, next you'll choose view all laboratory categories, then click the hyperlinks for medical laboratory services and test facilities. They also have links for testing services and lab equipment.

Quick replay, using ThomasNet can help you to increase your visibility, target your marketing efforts, and connect with potential clients in the healthcare industry. It is important to keep in mind that listing your business on ThomasNet is just one part of a comprehensive marketing strategy, and it is important to use a variety of channels and tactics to promote your business and attract new clients.

Here are a few labs below to help get started with partnerships.

- Spectracell Laboratories,
- Vibrant America,
- Oxford Biomedical Technologies,
- Boston Heart Diagnostics,
- E-Screen,
- Quest,
- LabCorp,
- KBMO Diagnostics,
- GetLabs,
- Ulta Lab Tests, (affiliate link, accepts HAS/FSA & earn commission from sales)
- Peekaboo,
- SneakPeek (affiliate link available)
- Alcat,
- Alletess,
- Beaumont,
- Cyrex,
- CirrusDX,
- Tetracore,

- *IgenX,*
- *True Health, (affiliate link)*
- *Natera,*

An important note to remember, any lab will accept collections and specimens as long as you can provide the physician's order. A contract is not required when dropping off the collections and specimens to your local labs and hospitals.

CHAPTER 48

The Advantages Of Using Fiverr

Using Fiverr to brand and market your business can provide several benefits. Fiverr offers a wide range of branding and marketing services, including logo design and all types of signage, website design or redesign, social media management, content creation, standard operating procedures and so much more. This can help you to find the right freelancer for your specific needs and budget.

Fiverr offers affordable pricing options, including many services that start at just $5. This can be a cost-effective way to access high-quality branding and marketing services without breaking your budget. Fiverr allows you to find the right freelancer for your specific needs and allows you to scale your branding and marketing efforts as needed. This can help you to stay flexible and adapt to changing market conditions.

Fiverr offers a range of tools and features that help to ensure quality and satisfaction, such as reviews, ratings, and dispute resolution. This can help you to find high-quality freelancers and ensure that your branding and marketing efforts are effective. Outsourcing branding and marketing tasks to freelancers on Fiverr can help you to save time and focus on other areas of your business. This can be especially beneficial if you have limited resources or are working on a tight schedule.

Quick replay, using Fiverr to brand and market your business can provide several benefits, including access to a wide range of services, cost-effective solutions, flexibility, high-quality services, and time savings. It is important to carefully vet freelancers and ensure that they have the necessary skills and expertise to help you achieve your branding and marketing goals.

Branding, marketing, and advertising are essential components of a successful business strategy because they help increase visibility, build credibility and establish a strong reputation in the marketplace. Effective branding helps make your business recognizable and

memorable to potential customers. By developing a distinctive visual identity and consistent messaging, you can create a strong brand that stands out from competitors and builds loyalty among customers.

Marketing and advertising efforts can help increase awareness of your business among potential customers. By targeting your ideal audience through various channels such as social media, email marketing, and paid advertising, you can increase your reach and generate more leads.

A strong brand and marketing strategy can help establish your business as a credible and trustworthy provider of mobile phlebotomy services. By sharing testimonials, showcasing expertise, and providing educational content, you can build trust with potential clients and position yourself as an authority in the field. A strong brand and reputation can encourage satisfied clients to refer their friends and family to your business, which can help generate new business without additional marketing expenses.

Quick replay, branding, marketing, and advertising are crucial components of any successful business strategy. By establishing a strong brand and implementing effective marketing tactics, you can increase visibility, build credibility, and attract more customers to your mobile phlebotomy business.

CHAPTER 49

Digital Marketing

There are several different ways to market your mobile phlebotomy business, depending on your target audience, budget, and goals.

Social media: Create a strong social media presence on platforms such as Facebook, Instagram, and LinkedIn. Share educational content, testimonials, and promotions to engage with potential clients and build brand awareness.

Paid advertising: Consider running targeted ads on social media or search engines to reach a wider audience. You can also advertise in local publications or sponsor relevant events or organizations.

Referral marketing: Encourage satisfied clients to refer their friends and family to your business by offering incentives or rewards for referrals.

Content marketing: Create educational blog posts, videos, or other content that positions you as an expert in the field and provides value to potential clients.

Email marketing: Build an email list and send regular newsletters or promotions to keep clients engaged and informed about your services.

Direct mail: Send targeted postcards or mailers to potential clients in specific geographic areas or demographic groups.

Community involvement: Get involved in local healthcare events, volunteer opportunities, or sponsorships to build relationships and increase visibility in the community.

SEO: Optimize your website and online listings for search engines to increase your visibility in relevant search results.

Remember to tailor your marketing

approach to your specific target audience and goals, and to track and analyze your results to make data-driven decisions about your marketing strategy.

CHAPTER 50

Standard Operating Procedures

Standard Operating Procedures (SOPs) are documented procedures that outline the steps involved in performing a specific task or process. You can get a freelancer on Fiverr to create them for you. SOPs ensure that all procedures are performed consistently and accurately by every team member, regardless of their level of experience. This can help to reduce errors and improve the quality of service.

SOPs can help to streamline procedures and reduce the time it takes to complete them. This can help to increase productivity and reduce costs. They provide a framework for training new employees, which can help to ensure that they receive consistent and accurate training. SOPs help to ensure that procedures are performed in compliance with legal and regulatory requirements. This can help to reduce the risk of legal and regulatory issues. SOPs can help to ensure that procedures are performed

safely and minimize the risk of injury or illness to both employees and clients.

Quick replay, having SOPs in place for a mobile phlebotomy business can help to ensure consistency, efficiency, proper training, compliance, and safety. It is important to review and update SOPs regularly to ensure that they remain relevant and effective.

CHAPTER 51

If I Can Do This, So Can You

Becoming a mobile phlebotomy and lab business owner can be challenging, but it's important to remember the reasons why you started your business in the first place. Whether it's a desire for independence, a passion for healthcare, or a commitment to providing quality service to your patients, these reasons can serve as a powerful motivator when things get tough.

It's also important to remember that success rarely happens overnight. Building a successful mobile phlebotomy business takes time, effort, and patience. It's normal to experience setbacks and challenges along the way, but these experiences can provide valuable learning opportunities that help you improve and grow your business.

To stay motivated, focus on your successes and celebrate your achievements, no matter how small. Surround yourself with supportive friends, family, and colleagues who can provide

encouragement and advice when you need it. And always keep your eye on your goals and your passion for your business, as these are the things that will sustain you through the ups and downs of entrepreneurship. Owning a mobile phlebotomy and lab business can be a rewarding and fulfilling career, and with determination, perseverance, and a commitment to excellence, you can achieve your dreams and build a business that you are proud of.

Playbook replay, Creating and growing a successful mobile phlebotomy business requires careful planning, dedication, and a commitment to providing high-quality service to your patients. By following best practices for business planning, branding, marketing, and customer service, you can build a strong reputation and attract a loyal customer base. Additionally, staying up-to-date on industry trends and investing in new technologies can help you stay ahead of the competition and provide the best possible service to your patients. With hard work, determination, and a focus on delivering exceptional value, you can build a thriving mobile phlebotomy business that serves your community and supports your financial goals.

CHAPTER 50

Government Resource Links

49 CFR, Part 40 Regulations

https://www.transportation.gov/odapc/part40

Health and Human Services Mandatory Guidelines for workplace testing

https://www.samhsa.gov/workplace/resources

Drug and Alcohol Testing Regulations for NRC

https://www.nrc.gov/reading-rm/doc-collections/cfr/part026/part026-0031.html

Certified Laboratories for Drug Testing

https://www.samhsa.gov/workplace/drug-testing-resources/certified-lab-list

State Survey Agencies (Clia Contact List) (Cms.Gov)

https://www.cms.gov/regulations-and-guidance/legislation/clia/downloads/cliasa.pdf

Clinical Laboratory Improvement Amendments

(CLIA) | CMS

https://www.cms.gov/regulations-and-guidance/legislation/clia

How to Enroll in Medicare Electronic Data Interchange | CMS

https://www.cms.gov/Medicare/Billing/ElectronicBillingEDITrans/EnrollInEDI

Introducing PECOS 2.0 | CMS

https://www.cms.gov/medicare/provider-enrollment-and-certification/introducing-pecos-20

National Provider Identifier Standard (NPI) | CMS

https://www.cms.gov/Regulations-and-Guidance/Administrative-Simplification/NationalProvIdentStand

CFR, Part 40.43 (Collection Sites, Forms Equipment and Supplies for DOT Drug Testing)

https://www.transportation.gov/odapc/part40/40-43

Approved Alcohol Screening Devices (ASD) Conforming Products List

https://www.transportation.gov/odapc/Approved-Screening-Devices-to-Measure-Alcohol

Approved Evidential Breath Testing Devices (EBT) Conforming Products List

https://www.transportation.gov/odapc/approved-evidential-breath-testing-devices

Office of Drug and Alcohol Policy and Compliance website

https://www.transportation.gov/odapc

Subscribe to ODAPC List Serve

https://www.transportation.gov/odapc/ListServe_Notices

Business and Marketing Resource Links

Writing your Business Plan (SBA Resource)

https://www.sba.gov/business-guide/plan-your-business/write-your-business-plan

Calculating your Startup costs (SBA Resource)

https://www.sba.gov/business-guide/plan-your-business/calculate-your-startup-costs

Small Business Administration website

https://www.sba.gov/

http://www.fiverr.com/s2/8ee9b52d7b

Home - Canva

https://www.canva.com/

https://www.ultalabtests.com/partners/kwanajones/affiliate/get-started

Video: How to set-up a Facebook Business Page

https://www.youtube.com/watch?v=Zl87ugrZSf0

Facebook Business Page Set-Up

https://www.facebook.com/business/tools/facebook-pages/get-started

Set-up a LinkedIn Company Page

https://business.linkedin.com/marketing-solutions/linkedin-pages

Step-by-Step instructions for creating a LinkedIn

Company Page

https://www.linkedin.com/help/lms/answer/a54 3852/create-a-linkedin-page?lang=en

Video: How to complete a LinkedIn Company Page

https://www.youtube.com/watch?v=-hnPA9a4PaU

WIX Logo Maker

https://www.wix.com/logo/maker

WIX website templates

https://www.wix.com/

Website Builder | Create a Free Website in Minutes - GoDaddy

https://www.godaddy.com/websites/website-builder

Wordpress website templates

https://wordpress.com/

Marketing Collateral Templates

https://www.vistaprint.com/

SEO Basics: How to Do SEO for Beginners (semrush.com)

https://www.semrush.com/blog/seo-basics/?kw=&cmp=US_SRCH_DSA_Blog_Core_BU_EN&label=dsa_pagefeed&Network=g&Device=c&utm_content=484020087345&kwid=dsa-1057183198995&cmpid=11769537497&agpid=117334831871&BU=Core&extid=23669721292&adpos=&gclid=EAIaIQobChMIptiHl4yj-AIVbmpvBB14ewEuEAAYAiAAEgJPNfD_BwE

Popl Digital Business Cards | All Digital Business Cards - Popl

https://popl.co/collections/all-products

Yelp Business Page Set-Up

https://business.yelp.com/

Video: Google My Business Listing Set Up

https://www.youtube.com/watch?v=KWZs5ITvzbw

Google Business Profile Get Started

https://support.google.com/business/answer/633

7413?hl=en

Blog Article: Ultimate Guide to Google My Business

https://blog.hubspot.com/marketing/google-my-business

Google Pay-Per-Click Ads Overview

https://ads.google.com/home/#!/

Features - EnGuard

https://www.enguard.com/features/

Our Features - eFax

https://www.efax.com/features

Regus | Serviced Office Space, Coworking & Virtual Offices

https://www.regus.com/en-us

Professional Liability Insurance Facts - Malpractice FAQs (cmfgroup.com)

https://www.cmfgroup.com/frequently-asked-questions/

Features To Make Customer Booking Easy & Memorable | Setmore

https://www.setmore.com/features

Client Management Software for Small Businesses | HoneyBook

https://www.honeybook.com/getstarted?utm_source=bing&utm_campaign=396260769&utm_medium=cpc&utm_content=e&utm_term=honeybook%20pricing&placement=1251244870324728&device=c&gclid=21a0c86f9f6c1e0e9280ac72497c93f8&gclsrc=3p.ds&msclkid=21a0c86f9f6c1e0e9280ac72497c93f8

Pulmolab.com

https://pulmolab.com/

Psychology Today: Health, Help, Happiness + Find a Therapist

https://www.psychologytoday.com/us